What You Need to Know About Getting in Shape: Tips & Strategies from 10 Top Trainers

United Print Publishers

DEDICATION

This book is dedicated to all of the incredible professionals and companies who took the time to submit content to this book. It has been a pleasure working with each of you, on the production of this book. The time you have all taken and the high quality content that you have all shared has truly gone above and beyond anything we could have ever expected when we first set out to publish this book. Thank you to everyone who made this possible.

DISCLAIMER

or physical condition. If you choose to follow any advice within this book, you do so of your own free will and accord, knowingly and voluntarily assuming all risks associated with such activities.

Facts and information are believed to be accurate at the time they were published in this book. All information provided is to be used for informational purposes only. Products and services described are only offered in jurisdictions where they may be legally offered. Information provided is not all-inclusive, and is limited to information that is made available. Such information should not be relied upon as all-inclusive or accurate.

You agree to hold UNITED PRINT PUBLISHERS, its owners, agents, and employees harmless from any and all liability for all claims for damages due to injuries, including attorney fees and costs, incurred by you or caused to third parties by you, arising out of the fitness and diet plans discussed in this book.

Testimonials, case studies, and examples within this book are unverified results that have been forwarded to us by the interviewees featured in this book, and may not reflect the typical reader's experience, may not apply to the average person, and are not intended to represent or guarantee that anyone will achieve the same or similar results. You should always perform due diligence and not take such results at face value. We are not responsible for any errors or omissions in typical results information supplied to us by third parties.

CONTENTS

ACKNOWLEDGMENTS

Shape Up Fitness & Wellness Consulting
Healthy Now, Healthy For Life, LLC
Pilates of Eastlake
Joe Martin Fitness LLC
Life Fitness Academy
Barry's Bootcamp
Steps Inc.
Innovative fitness
Poise Health & Fitness
Center-Fit

Thank you to the following fitness experts who without their contributions and support this book would not have been written: Michael Anders, Robert Lekan, Lariesa Bernick, Joe Martin, Terry Barga, Derrick Sobotka, Irv Rubenstein, Danny Kaczmarek, Crystal Dawn Potter, and Steve & Tori Bradford.

INTRODUCTION

If you've ever spent any amount of time strolling through the "Fitness & Nutrition" books section, at your local book store, you've probably noticed one thing: There sure are a lot of books on the subject of losing weight and eating healthy. While this large amount of information on the subject may seem like a good thing, it could also be the one thing that keeps you from taking action towards your personal fitness and nutrition goals.

As you're probably aware, the fitness and nutrition industry is a multi-billion dollar industry. There are thousands upon thousands of people who rely on you to buy the next fitness book, exercise gadget, or DVD that hits the store shelves or the late night TV airwaves. Unfortunately, in this profit-driven world known as the fitness and nutrition industry, one priority gets lost: Getting real results for the end-user. You see, if one of these multi-million dollar companies actually produced a gadget or DVD that enabled everyone to be in the best shape of their lives forever, you wouldn't need to buy their products anymore - and that's exactly what they don't want to happen!

So what does this mean for you? Should you just throw in the towel and give up on any and all information out there? Of course not. You do, however, need to be more selective in where you get your information from.

The goal of this book was to interview real personal trainers who really train clients each and every day of their professional lives. When we produced this book, we set out to find real world experts and that's exactly what we got. Our biggest challenge was getting these personal trainers to break away from their busy schedules of training their clients, so that they could actually share their advice in this book. The trainers who have contributed to this book "walk the walk", and the content they've provided, in the following chapters, reflects their true knowledge and expertise. So, without further ado, we present to you, the real world expert interviews!

WHAT YOU NEED TO KNOW ABOUT GETTING IN SHAPE

INTERVIEW WITH MICHAEL ANDERS

1 SUCCEEDING MENTALLY FIRST

Shape Up Fitness & Wellness Consulting is one of the leading personal training companies in Charlotte, NC in training quality and customer experience. We accomplish this by having a team of passionate trainers and employees that deeply care about creating an environment of caring, learning and passion for fitness. This environment empowers all of us, owner, employee and client to accomplish goals and enrich lives in a way that goes beyond fitness and training. Our motto: Shape Up Fitness & Wellness Consulting - Transforming one Life at Time!

Is it better to exercise every part of the body on the same day, or it better to focus on different muscle groups on different days? Please explain why one is better than the other.

That really depends on how often a person is working out in a week. If a client trains 2-3 days a week focusing on certain muscle groups would be wasted time and she/he would not get the biggest bang for her buck. The goal is to get the most results possible, therefore you work the whole body if the client trains 2-3 days a week. If someone lifts 4 days a week you use a split routine like (Upper/Lower Body). We do not really recommend lifting more than 4 days a week but rather do some cross-training instead.

Should women lift weights if they don't want to get bulky looking? If yes, how can they lift weights and not get that bulky/masculine look?

Absolutely yes. All of our female clients lift heavy at some point unless it is medically contraindicated. None of them look masculine. Women do not have the hormone levels necessary to look like guys and even if they build muscle more easily than others, it is a transformation and does not happen overnight.

In order to look like a bodybuilder you have to train like one. No woman lifting 2-3 days a week, even really heavy, will look like a dude. Instead she will gain a toned, feminine, aesthetic body. Every training comes in phases and if you rotate your training properly, changing from lower weights and higher repetitions to heavier weights and less repetitions the body will develop in a balanced healthy way that promotes fitness, aesthetics and health.

Is it true that some people naturally lose weight faster than others? Why or why not is this the case?

There are different body types, we have ectomorph, mesomorph and endomorph body types. Ectomorph body types are usually taller and really lean. They can eat without gaining weight. The endomorph body type is on the other end of the spectrum, shorter, stouter and more prone to gaining weight, these people have to really watch their nutrition.

The mesomorph body type gains muscle mass more easily and is leaner than the endomorph body type but not quite as lean as the ectomorph. Only 3 % of the population fall into the extreme corners of body types. We usually are a mix between the three types. Gender plays a role as well: Men usually lose weight faster than women do their increased lean muscle mass/ lb. body mass.

What precautions should seniors take into consideration, when starting a new exercise program?

Always get a checkup by your primary care physician first. If you have been sedentary for a while you might not be aware what impact exercise can have on possible conditions like hypertension, hypercholesterolemia, arthritis, etc. By working closely with your health care professionals you will have more fun training and most likely less injuries. I would always recommend working with a trainer in the beginning, at least for a short period of time to get a well-structured training plan that takes your goals and needs into consideration.

Is it typical for a personal trainer to ask their clients to sign a contract? If so, what are some standard contract lengths and terms?

That strongly varies from company to company. I don't believe in clients having to sign away their life. Instead they work with us on a monthly basis. But signing up for big packages is quite common in the personal training world. If I would look for a trainer to work with I would ask for the following:

1. Initial consultation to meet the trainer
2. Ask for a starter package or a money back guarantee (30 days) if you don't like it.
3. Don't be afraid to ask for a different trainer if you are not comfortable with yours.

If someone enjoys drinking alcohol in moderation, how often can they indulge without feeling guilty or undoing all the progress they made with their trainer?

That is a dangerous question. "Moderation" is different for everyone. Initially I would recommend not drinking for 30 days to get everything on track. Later, one glass of wine / day (3-5 oz.) if the nutrition is right on track is not a problem if people don't start eating more at the same time. Inhibition is the first thing to go when drinking alcohol, therefore it is better to limit it to 1-2 glasses per week.

What can people do if they "plateau" and stop seeing results from their workout routine?

Every body gets used to what it is doing. Your training should change every 4 weeks. Mix up the exercises, change the intensity, breaks and the volume. Mix in some high intensity interval training to increase your metabolism. As an example: If you have been lifting weights for 3 sets and 15 Repetitions with short breaks, drop down to 3-4 sets with 5-8 repetitions with longer breaks (60-120s). Your body will wake up for sure!

Is it true that genetics or body physiology make it impossible for some people to get in shape?

No, unless someone has a medical condition everyone can be healthy, fit and in shape. It might be more difficult for different body types but it is never impossible. They key factors for being fit and in shape are the following:

1. Sleep: sleep lets us recover. If we do not get enough sleep our hormone levels are off and weight loss is near impossible.

2. Nutrition: "We are what we eat!" Eat healthy minimally processed food and you will most likely lose weight.

3. Lifestyle: Be as active as you can. You might exercise 6 days a week for an hour. Well the week has 144 hours so that is not that much. Move a lot when you are not exercising and the fat is melting off.

4. Exercise: Train smart not hard. For years we thought that the more is better. Lift three days a week and do some high intensity interval training 3 days a week. You spend relatively little time in the gym and you have huge benefits.

What is the "fat burning zone" that trainers often refer to?

The fat burning zone was defined as the heart rate range that burns primarily fat. Research indicates that high intensity interval training or even just more intense steady state aerobic exercises burns a whole lot more calories overall and in fat than the fat burning zone in a smaller time frame. Considering the time pressure people are in nowadays, training needs to be effective. Training in the fat burning zone for hours to have the same results that you could have in 20-30 min with a higher intensity workout does not make any sense. Especially since interval training increases your metabolism considerably for a couple of hours after you are actually done training.

Do people really lose muscle as they get older? If so, how much muscle do they lose on average, and can anything be done to slow down this process?

It seems that we lose about 1% per year of muscle mass after the age of 30. Make sure to include a strenuous strength exercise regimen into your regular workout routines. Make sure that the protein intake is high enough. Beyond that older people respond really well to a resistance training with strength gains that are equivalent to that of young adults. For most people the loss of muscle mass is due to their sedentary lifestyle. They would only experience the effects of aging once they are highly trained. Most individuals do not train at those levels. If there are no medical restrictions training at a high intensity (heavy weights, 80% of 1RM) has huge benefits.

Is it safe to workout first thing in the morning, on an empty stomach?

That depends on you. Some people do not function well without food first thing, others throw up if they eat before their morning workouts. Test it out and see what works for you. If you don't want to get up too early mix some Gatorade with some water for your more intense workouts. This helps you avoid hitting the wall.

Is it true that it's good to have a "cheat day" where people can eat whatever they want once a week? Why is this a good or bad idea?

I am not a big fan of a cheat day. Because a cheat day often becomes a "cheat two days" and then a whole week. It seems to be hard to get back on the wagon and you can really destroy all of your progress in one day if you go all out. We recommend to have one cheat meal out of ten good ones, if you need it. Please don't make it a typical Thanksgiving Dinner though.

HOW TO CONTACT US

Michael Anders

Owner, Head Trainer of Shape Up Fitness & Wellness Consulting

Website: www.charlottepersonaltrainer.org

Email: michael@charlottepersonaltrainer.org

Phone: 704 777 3743

2 HOW TO LIVE A HEALTHY LIFESTYLE

The emphasis is on balance, integrated and holistic viewpoint of health and wellness. Health is not meant to be just physical, but through mental and emotional wellbeing by employing a network of trained and certified practitioners of various modalities to help the client reach their ultimate state of wellbeing.

If someone eats very healthy, and they have an active lifestyle, do they still need to workout? Why or why not?

They do need to work out for several reasons. Working out not only helps being physically healthy, it helps with movement, daily living as well as helping their mental and emotional states. When a person works out, they are able to handle better higher levels of stress without detriment to their own health. They are able to help move through their body in a pain free state.

As many people today deal with issues of being in a sitting, lethargic and cramped work environment, the mental and sometimes emotional stress they encounter at their job forces their body to tighten and stiffen, causing imbalances and physical issues. Pain inhibits movement. Lack of movement or improper movement causes a person to remain more in a stationary state. Lack of activity wears on the mental and emotional well-being on a person helping to cause them to create situations, (poor eating habits, depression, etc), further spiraling them in to an unhealthy situation. Working out is one part, but an easier part for a client to do for themselves by themselves.

How can a personal trainer help a client, with regard to nutrition?

A well informed trainer often meets with a client more often than a doctor or most other health professional. A well informed trainer can help talk with a client, monitor their eating habits, track their results more often and be able to give them feedback and better direction more immediately then most health professionals which are seen perhaps once to twice a month or even year.

What are some examples of foods that people think are good for them, but they're really not, and why are these foods actually not healthy?

Most people focus on low fat foods, especially when they are prepackaged and prepared foods. Salad dressings, cookies and other foods trick most people in to thinking they are eating something they enjoy without doing much harm to their actual bodies. Most that are low fat are replaced with chemicals or sugars to mimic the flavors they crave, which doesn't create a better health, just shifts the unhealthy calories and intake in another direction, such as being addicted to diet drinks, sugar or other substances.

What are some factors that impact people's metabolism?

Blood sugar and the lack awareness of what people eat. Most people are unaware of what they eat and why they are eating them. The cycle that tends to be seen is when they feel low, depressed or having a bad day they tend to mindlessly eat. When that happens, they tend to over eat, snack on packaged food filled with sugar or poly saturated fat which makes them feel better and also spikes their blood sugar.

This produces a temporary high if good feelings and spikes the blood sugar. When the blood sugar spikes, the body produces insulin to help deal with the intake of sugar.

When the sugar intake in consistently too high, as tends to happen with a processed carb heavy diet, the body can't produce enough insulin to deal with it and it becomes insulin resistant. This adds to a higher fat in the body, slower metabolism and predispositions people to become pre-diabetic or diabetic. Also more people tend to pay attention to the bigger words or not taking the time to understand labels on food, causing them not be able to understand what is and what isn't healthy.

Is there any true benefit to warming up, cooling down, or stretching before or after exercising? If there is, why are these things important?

There are benefits for all of them. Warming up not only increases your range of motion, prepares your body for a workout by not only increasing your blood flow but with increasing the sensory systems of your body. It also helps to activate your mind and puts it on alert to be aware of how you are using your body and to be aware of how it feels when working out. This does not mean normal static stretching of just holding a stretch through a held position, this is more in terms of dynamic stretching and allowing the body to move through a motion.

Cooling down and stretching I tend to put in the same. This does not mean they are the same. Cooling down can mean breathing techniques, stretching, ice baths and so on.

This allows the body to begin the repair stage and rejuvenation of the body. It allows the heart rate to slow down and for any muscles/joints that need to prepare to be opened can at that time.

Once someone begins working out with a personal trainer, what goes on during the sessions?

That is pretty much up to the client and the trainer. Every trainer has his or her formula that works for them and what they perceive with their client. Warming up, dynamic stretching, stabilization exercises, balance, core, strength, cardio, plyometrics, boxing, tai chi, Qi gong etc... Every trainer has their method. What should typically happens is a greeting, some short induction on how the client is feeling, any issues they have going on, a quick review of what of a plan for during the session, the actual session and possibly some sort of cool down if there is time or if the client requests it.

How can people accurately determine how many calories they burn during a workout?

The best way these days is a calorie counter. Several companies have them, many with a heart rate monitor with an estimated calories burned. This varies per model. It will give a good ratio or idea, but exact counts can be hard to figure out. The ones given on a cardio machine are rarely accurate, the best for a personal count is something that you wear throughout a workout and has some personal information about your body.

What should someone look for in a good health club/gym?

What should be decided before someone ever looks at a health club is to decide what they need it for. If it is mainly to do cardio and maybe some crunches, minimal equipment should be looked for. If it is something more specific or the client needs a variety, making sure there is a wide variety of options or goes in the vein of what the specific goals and needs are. What should be looked for is a clean gym, functioning equipment, friendly staff. Make sure all areas are looked at and you feel comfortable with it all.

How can people prevent joint injuries or sore joints when lifting weights?

First of all, start slowly. If you haven't been to a gym from a few months to never, you should start slowly. Your body can't go from 0 to 100 in a 6 seconds, it needs to be warmed up. If you are unsure about things, this would be a good time to start with a trainer to understand basics with form, understand with how stable they are in their body and a general course of action.

If your body is out of alignment it will not function correctly. If you add weight and speed to a dysfunctioning body, you will just exasperate the issues and make them worse. Making sure you move correctly is the first step, then moving correctly consistently is the next.

What types of scheduling commitments are customary, when hiring a personal trainer? In other words, do people normally take things one week at a time or are they typically asked to schedule several weeks at a time with their trainer?

Every trainer is different as each client. It is typical to schedule week by week, with sometime during the previous week the next week's session/s will be decided. Some clients who are about to have a crazy hectic week will want to schedule a few weeks in advanced, but that is up to the client and what they need.

What if someone is completely out of shape? What's the safest approach for getting started?

Slowly. Many clients like to jump in to the thick of things and start off hard core, which tends to be the biggest mistake. Start slowly but consistently. Make sure workouts are planned and kept. Even if it is 45 minutes of walking on a treadmill, it is a start. The biggest thing is to move slowly and consistently, if you stumble one day, then make sure you start again the next day and not to try and double your efforts.

Add changes slowly, one or two per every two to three weeks. They are supposed to be meaningful changes, they won't happen overnight. And that is the other thing, to be safe, you have to be patient. Every client can make their goal, but if they don't understand that this is a slow process and it won't happen overnight, then they will easily get frustrated or they will try and push themselves way beyond their limit, feel like they are failing and quit. Keep things in perspective and look at the big picture. It will happen.

HOW TO CONTACT US

Rob Lekan

Owner of Healthy Now, Healthy For Life, LLC

PersonalTrainerRobChi@gmail.com

twitter @positiveinlife

INTERVIEW WITH LARIESA BERNICK

3 TIPS FOR BEST RESULTS

- ACE certified Personal Trainer, Group Fitness Instructor
 - Balanced Body Certified Pilates Instructor
- 2 Nationally sold fitness DVD's
- Expert guest speaker on Comcast Cable television
 - Featured Business of the Month in My Hometown Magazine - Author of* Your Beautiful Body: Using Pilates at Home to Overcome Weight Loss Obstacles* (2011)

What are the best types of exercises for getting the fastest results in the shortest period of time?

Exercises that burns calories quickly while boosting your muscle mass will fire up your metabolism and melt off the fat! It is possible to get better results with an effective 10-minute workout than a longer one. Do explosive exercises such as jumping jacks and squat jumps. Alternate these types of high-energy workouts with sprints instead of long walks. Don't forget frequent short breaks! And you will be in shape in less time than a longer, traditional workout.

Is it true that people with diabetes have a harder time losing weight? If so, why is this the case?

People who have diabetes absolutely can lose weight, and should. It is a delicate balance in keeping your blood sugar stable while you exercise, as exercise may cause a drop in blood sugar. Both type 1 and type 2 diabetes ultimately lead to high blood sugar levels, so losing even 5-10% of your weight can significantly help to lower blood sugar, and possibly even allow you to come off of insulin. Just make sure you let your doctor help keep your blood sugar levels stable as you go through this very rewarding process.

If someone hasn't worked out in years, how should they get started in the safest way possible?

Any person starting an exercise program should plan specific days, say 2 or 3 days of the week that they intend to exercise. Overdoing it too soon is the number one reason I see people fail to reach their goals. Allow yourself to start slow by taking a day to walk, and another day or two to do strength training exercises. After a week or two, add in another walking day. This gives the body time to adjust and recover. The same process should occur for the diet so that too many changes aren't made at once. After all, being healthy is a lifestyle change that can't be accomplished overnight. With time you will be running instead of walking and lean and healthy! All because you took the time to do things the right way.

What are some of the most common myths about building muscle?

One of those most common things I hear from women is that they are concerned that they will have giant muscles if they lift heavy weights. Nothing could be farther from the truth! Using a resistance that is challenging during strength training will not only create sculpted muscles, it will shrink the body by making everything firmer. Have you ever noticed that the leanest women in the gym are the ones lifting the weights, not the ones glued to the cardio machines? That's because strength training will firm up the body while creating lean toned muscles.

Aim to do resistance exercises twice per week, and lift heavy enough that the muscles become fatigues after 10-15 repetitions. You would have to do SOOOO much more than this to build muscle mass, and most women have that result anyway. Men can create hypertrophy (building muscle mass) easier than us girls can because their higher levels of testosterone fuel the muscles to gain lean mass. So don't worry ladies! Pick up those dumbbells and bring on the lean figure!

Do people need exercise equipment to get in shape?

People definitely do not need exercise equipment to get into shape. It is absolutely possible to become fit without buying expensive machines. In fact, it's actually unnecessary. You can get a complete full body workout by doing body weight exercises in your own home such as push ups, crunches, squats, planks. Then take walks outside to get all the cardio you need.

If going outside isn't your favorite, you can create a cardio, sculpting workout by adding jumping jack or squat jump intervals to your in-home routine. I also love having exercise tubing to add resistance to exercises. It takes zero space and less than $10, yet it is like having a full gym in your house. Skip the expensive and unnecessary equipment; you can do better with a basic exercise band and your living room floor.

Is coffee bad for someone who's trying to lose weight or get in shape?

Coffee is not bad for someone trying to lose weight. In fact, caffeine acts as a stimulant which increases the heart rate. This elevation in heart rate can actually improve you workout by giving you that little extra edge to actually work harder and burn more calories! Just make sure you stay hydrated, as caffeine is a diuretic. For every 8 oz. of coffee you consume, you should drink an extra glass of water, in addition to rehydrating after your workout. So go ahead and have that little jolt of coffee; it may just fuel your workout to that much more effective!

Is aerobic walking as healthy as jogging or running?

Aerobic walking is absolutely as good as jogging or running, and a lot easier on your knees. You will burn about 80% of the calories that you would if you were running as long as you keep the pace brisk. Here is a good rule of thumb... use the "talk test" to make sure you are working out effectively: if you can carry on a conversation with your friend while you are walking, then you aren't walking fast enough! You should barely be able to carry on a broken conversation in between breaths.. then you know you are walking in a way that will be just about as effective as jogging.

Can someone still lose weight if they split their workouts throughout the day?

Yes! You can absolutely split your workouts into little "mini" sessions. Studies have shown that doing 10 minute sessions throughout the day is just as effective as working out in one long session. Aim to get your full workout time in by creating sneaky opportunities to exercise. For example, park your car on the other end of the lot and briskly walk to your office. Climb the stairs a few times on your lunch break. Do pushups against the kitchen counter and squats while you are cooking. Voila!!! You will have already managed your daily quota of exercise without ever planning a trip to the gym!

HOW TO CONTACT US

Lariesa Bernick

Owner and founder of Pilates of Eastlake

Website: www.pilatesofeastlake.com

Phone: 619-213-2181

4 PREPARING FOR YOUR WORKOUT

Joe Martin Fitness LLC is a fitness company that believes in constant improvement, getting results, and caring for their clients. We specialize in fat loss through fitness boot camps, on-line virtual personal training, and nutrition and fitness books. We have won awards for being the healthiest place to exercise as well as having the healthiest trainer.

What is the correct way to breathe when working out?

This may sound ridiculous to some people, but as a trainer I have to frequently remind people to breathe period! Proper breathing is an often overlooked skill, but can really improve your overall fitness performance and enjoyment. There is an old saying in the fitness world "Control your breathing before it controls you."

If you are not conscious of your breathing it can affect how well you can perform/complete your exercise program. There are different breathing techniques that I recommend for cardiovascular training, resistance training, and stretching. To get the most out of your cardiovascular exercise, belly breathing is the best method. The easiest way to think about proper belly breathing is to breathe in so your belly rises and falls, not just your chest.

If you have ever got a side cramp while running, you know how painful it can be. To help avoid that awful sensation, practice breathing in deeply and then breathing out every other time your left foot hits the ground. Not only will this help you avoid side cramps, but also because it will help you get in a nice rhythm. This may sound like a weird tip, but it works.

These side stitches are basically spasms of the diaphragm that running can cause because it makes the organs attached to the diaphragm jump up and down. You put a much larger strain on the organs attached to the diaphragm when you breathe out when your right foot hits. The organs on the left side are much smaller, so there is less strain.

When you are doing resistance training, whether it is with your own body or with weights, you need to breathe out when you are exerting force and breathe in as you lower the load back down. When doing a pushup, you would breathe in as you lower yourself to the ground and forcefully breathe out as you push yourself back up for example. Think of it as your breath propelling you away from the ground.

When stretching, you should be breathing nice and steady throughout the whole stretch. If you are looking to increase the stretch as you go, try to stretch a little further as you breathe out. How can people tell if they're doing enough exercise or exercising intensely enough? A good way to check if you are exercising hard enough is to use the Karvonen method to determine your target heart rate. Here are the equations you need:

Max heart rate= 220-age

Target heart rate= ((Max heart rate - resting heart rate)) x % intensity + resting heart rate

You would then figure out the range you need to stay in. For prolonged, lower intensity exercise like a long jog would be 60% intensity, while higher intensity exercise like a sprint would be closer to 90% intensity. For those of you like myself with arithmophobia (fear of math) you can use a much simpler test called Perceived Rate of Exertion (PRE). It is basically a scale of 6-20 with 6 being no exertion, 13 being somewhat hard, 15 is hard, 19 is extremely hard, to 20 being maximal exertion AKA "I will die if I keep this up." Then you match up your intensity with the levels discussed above.

Then there are a few old fashioned, not quite as scientific ways to tell if you are exercising intensely enough.

-Did you break a sweat? Usually an indication that you are not working hard enough, although temperature can play a factor either way on this one.

-Can you hold a normal conversation? If so, you need to pick it up a little.

-Are you getting results? Are you losing inches/body fat/ and or weight? If you are not seeing results it is time to increase the intensity.

-Are you doing the same workout you were doing 3 months ago? If you are running the same distance in the same amount of time or lifting the same weight you were 3 months ago, it is time to make it harder.

How important is flexibility, when it comes to getting in shape? Why is this important?

I believe that the true fountain of youth lies in staying strong and flexible, so flexibility is absolutely crucial. There are several reasons why flexibility is important.

-Keeps you free from injury while exercising as well as when doing everyday tasks

-Improves posture and keeps you from that slumped over desk worker look that can lead to back problems

-Improves sports and athletic performance

-Makes exercise more effective because you are able to go through the full range of motion during movement

-Helps improve circulation to the muscles being stretched

-Helps improve muscle coordination and balance, making exercise easier and safer

Do minors typically need to get the permission of an adult or guardian, if they want to work with a personal trainer? If so, how does this work?

Minors absolutely need permission from an adult or guardian before starting any kind of exercise program with a trainer. Not only do they need permission from a legal stand point, but it is also very helpful to the trainer. Not very many kids know their complete health history (injuries, surgeries, allergies, etc...), which is an absolutely crucial part of any program.

Youth fitness is a very fast growing segment of the fitness world, with over $4 billion being spent on personal training and coaching of kids under 18 every year. It is a great trend and I hope to see it continue to grow and grow. But I would advise any parent getting their children into a fitness program to really research and find out who is the most qualified person or persons to help their kids.

Just like any sport or activity, if they get the wrong coach/trainer it can sour them for life on exercise. Definitely not something this country needs, considering the obesity rates among children. Every trainer is a little different, but typically the parent or guardian would just need to sign a waiver and healthy history questionnaire to get started. If there is not cause to consult a physician, then the child is okayed to exercise. Some trainers require a little more in depth process, some a little more but this is the typical process.

How will a trainer know what program is right for their client?

At the beginning of any training relationship, the trainer will find out through conversation or a health history form what goals the client has in mind. It is then up to the trainer to come up with a game plan that is suitable to that individual's goals, health history, preferences, and time commitment. It is very important for the client to interview prospective trainers before hiring them. Here are a few things to look into:

Education-Not an absolute must, but a degree in a related field (exercise physiology, exercise science, health promotion, etc...) does show a certain level of commitment to their profession.

Experience-An experienced trainer will have methods that have been proven in the field over the years and not just a workout that looks good on paper.

Certifications-Look for someone who is certified through an accredited organization (ACE, ACSM, NSCA are all good options) that requires continuing education.

Specialty-Every trainer has an area or a few select areas they really excel in. Whether it is a population (women, older adults, athletes, etc...) or an outcome (fat loss, muscle gain, race time), find a trainer that has a niche that is in line with your goals.

Referrals-Ask your friends, family, co-workers, or anyone you know who has a trainer what they think about them. This is often the best way to find a trainer you will be happy with.

Personality-This is one that is often overlooked, but is very important. If you are the type of person who bristles when someone yells at you, make sure you aren't hiring Jillian Michaels Jr.

After you go through this process, the client needs to put complete faith in their trainer. That is not to say the client should never question anything the trainer says or feel free to ask questions. It just means, now that you know what the trainer is all about you can feel comfortable in the knowledge the trainer has your best interest in mind. Your comfort level and your results will increase as your trust in your trainer rises as well. The perfect exercise program always involves open lines of communications through both parties.

For people who are always tired, won't working out make them feel like they have even less energy?

Being too tired to work out is a huge barrier for many people. The number one most important thing you can do when you think you are too tired to exercise, is to just get started. Sounds simple right? Some of the best workouts I have ever had in my life started with me thinking at a workout was the last place I ever wanted to be. Your body was built to move.

When you are sedentary, your energy levels being to drop. The body is an amazing machine that adapts to every situation you put it through. When you don't move or exercise for long periods of time, your body takes that as a signal that you do not need extra energy to do anything else. You now have just enough energy to sit 8 hours at work, then come home and sit 3 hours on the couch until it is bed time. But this phenomenon works both ways.

When you being to move more, exercise on a regular basis, and do the things your body was created to do your energy levels will sky rocket! It is a lot like life, just show up. Make it to the workout, start moving around a little, stretching, breaking a light sweat, etc... and the next thing you know you will have got in your workout and you will feel so much better. This workout does not have to be a 2 hour weight lifting session or a 13 mile run. You will be amazed at what a 20-30 minute brisk walk at lunch time will do for you, especially if that walk is replacing the sedentary lunch you normally participate in.

One tip that helps me is to always have my exercise clothes/equipment ready and with me at all times. You never know when you might get a break in your schedule and you will get the opportunity to exercise. Also, if you find things constantly getting in the way (work, kids, errands) after work, start exercising first thing in the morning. We have a 5:30am class and it is by far the most popular one we offer. Sounds ridiculous doesn't it? But that hour is what we call the No Excuses Hour.

There are no doctor's appointments or T-ball games that early in the morning. These are not morning people per se that attend that class. These are people who value their health and know that if it does not get done first thing in the morning, it will not happen. Then it will still be early in the morning, your workout is over, and you are energized and ready to take on the challenges of the day.

What are the benefits of hiring a personal trainer over just buying some DVDs that feature personal trainers?

Having a trainer eliminates two of the biggest stumbling blocks from people not reaching their goals: not being held accountable and getting injured. Accountability is one of the most important things for any exercise plan. What is going to make you show up for that workout when you are tired, sore, and just plain old don't feel like working out?

The DVD does not care what you do as long as you keep him properly dusted so he can spin contentedly in your DVD player. Your trainer on the other hand is not going to be so understanding. Trainers care about you getting results, it's why we do what we do. And we know that if you don't show up consistently, you are not going to get results.

There is nothing like an injury to make you never want to work out again. That is why having a trainer is very important, to help you prevent injury. There are three main things that contribute to injuries: Improper warm-up, improper form, and improper progression. A proper warm-up will prepare you mentally and physically for the rigors of the workout to help decrease injuries and increase performance.

Improper form will not only lead to injury, but also keep you from getting the most out of your workouts. Following an improper progression is a very common way people get hurt. Whether it is lifting too much too soon or running too far too soon, trying to do exercises your body is not prepared to handle is a sure fire way to get injured.

How much of a say should the client have in determining which exercises they do?

Clients should always have a say in what they will be doing, to a point. The main goal is to keep showing up for your workouts. Consistency is an absolute must to any successful exercise program. If a trainer comes up with the greatest program in the world, but the client hates every bit of it and never comes back, what good is that program?

On the other hand, the trainer is the expert in this subject matter.

Most people will choose the path of least resistance when it comes to most things. With exercise, it is literally the path with the least resistance (weight). Clients need to be pushed, they need to be challenged, but it also needs to be on their pace and level. With the huge variety of exercises out there, there is always a way to create a program that fits both the client's needs and the trainer's expectations.

Is it a good idea for someone to workout if they have a cold?

The general rule of the thumb I use for my clients is, if the cold is above the neck you are good but anything below the neck and you should not exercise. Exercise has actually been shown to not only help prevent colds, but studies have shown that people who exercise with a cold report feeling better than people who did not. The two main things to remember overall though are this: Listen to your body first.

If your body is telling you not to exercise, take a day off. You will not derail your whole exercise program by missing a day here and there. If there is ever any doubt, consult your doctor first because too much exercise when you are sick can make your condition worse.

Is it better to perform cardio before or after lifting weights or should cardio be done on a completely different day?

Here is my very scientific answer to that question, it depends. It depends on which one you hate the most and it depends on your schedule/how many days you have to exercise. There has been very little research to prove that one way or the other is a better method. So I would recommend you do whatever one you hate the most first and get it out of the way. This will greatly increase your chances of getting both done, rather than skipping out on whatever you are supposed to do second.

If I had to choose, I would recommend doing cardio and weights on different days if you have the time. That way you can go into both modes of exercise with full intensity.
But a more efficient and effective way is to combine cardio with strength training, through circuit training.

As an example, you would set up a circuit of 10 exercises alternating cardio with resistance training. Do each exercise for 40 seconds, rest 20 seconds, and then move onto the next exercise. Go through the entire list 2 times and you got a very fast and efficient workout in.

When people first start exercising, why do they sometimes gain weight initially?

This phenomenon is one of the main reasons I have encouraged my clients to quit seeing the scale as the only gauge of progress. A much more accurate way to see how you are progressing is to see how many inches you have lost, how your clothes are fitting, or body fat percentage lost. The scale can go up or down 5-10 pounds in one day! There are typically two main reasons I see for this weight gain.

The first is nothing to worry about, while the second needs to be addressed. The first culprit in this initial weight gain is water retention. This what happens to a lot of people when they start a strength training program. What you are doing when you are lifting weight is actually tearing them down while you exercise.

The process of your body building the muscles while you are at rest is when the magic actually happens. That is why you don't want to lift weights using the same muscles on back to back days. You have to give the body time to repair itself. This tearing down process makes the muscles inflamed. With this inflammation comes increased water retention and then the accompanying freak out when the scale goes up even after a lot of hard work.

The second reason the scale can go up when people first start working out is increased caloric intake. This especially occurs with resistance training because it really gets your metabolism revving, which increases your appetite. You cannot out exercise a bad diet. I have my clients keep a food journal, so they can see in black and white what they have been eating.

The rule with the food journal is, "If you bite it, you write it." Everything that has calories that you take in has to be recorded. It is a very eye opening experience to a lot of my clients who have never kept track. Use that food journal as a road map to figure out if it is the nutrition that needs to be assessed or something else. The scale is a fickle mistress, don't trust her.

If someone has a job where they don't move around a lot, what can they do to increase their activity during the day, when they're not working out?

Sedentary jobs are a big reason we have such an obesity epidemic in this country. A study out of UNC Wilmington found that people who began sedentary jobs put on 18 pounds over an 8 month period after starting the job. I have a question for you. Have you ever seen an overweight fidgeter?

Look at that annoying guy in your meeting who looks like he is working an old sewing machine in hyper drive the way he is tapping his foot. Usually a wiry guy. How about the lady who just can't seem to sit still? Fairly thin right? I think there is a lesson in there. Movement is the key to weight loss, so move more! Tapping your foot burns calories, pacing burns calories, even flicking a pin top up and down burns calories.

For true fidgeters it is usually second nature to fidget, but for normal people it takes a conscious effort. Find something that can help you burn a few extra calories. Walk to your co-worker's office down the hall, rather than e-mailing her. Stand up at least once an hour and do some kind of movement. You can burn around 100 calories and hour just by standing as opposed to sitting.

More and more people are even using desks that allow you to stand as you work. If you burned an extra 50 calories a day, you would lose about 5 pounds of fat per year. An extra 100 calories a day and you would lose 10 pounds of fat per year. Not too bad for a little extra effort.

HOW TO CONTACT US

Joe Martin

Owner of Joe Martin Fitness LLC

Website: http://www.JoeMartinFitness.com

Email: info@HuntsvilleBootCamp.com

Phone: 256.468.7146

INTERVIEW WITH TERRY BARGA

5 TRAINING LIKE A PROFESSIONAL

Life Fitness Academy is a holistic group of personal trainers, nutrition specialists, and fitness coaches. We believe that nutrition plays a vital role along with your fitness. We want the opportunity to show you how it has influenced us and how we can impact our community. We at Life Fitness Academy believe that our body, mind, spirit are all parts of our wellbeing. We believe whole health is a journey that should focus on every area of your life: spiritual, physical, and psychological. We have been where you are and love helping people out of that place and into whole health.

Why do people say, "Breakfast is the most important meal of the day"? Is there any truth in this?

When you eat isn't as important as what you eat. If your choices are to eat a donut or don't eat breakfast, don't eat breakfast. Eating something like that will take up to 48 hours to digest and because it takes so much energy to digest, it can leave you feeling more tired than if you skipped it. Concentrate more on giving your body the proper fuel to have energy for your day.

How can someone do resistance training if they don't own weights or belong to a gym?

You can easily use resistance bands in your home. You can find bands at most sporting goods stores and you can loop it around things in the room and do a variety of exercises. You have less chance of injuring yourself using a resistance band without supervision than with weights. Almost any moves with weights can be done with a resistance band.

Is it true that stress makes people gain weight? What is the truth, if any, behind this?

Cortisol is known as the stress hormone and is produced by the adrenal gland when you are stressed. It helps to support normal glucose metabolism, blood pressure levels, insulin release, immune function and inflammation levels, which means it can have some positive effects. When it's released in small amounts, cortisol can help you quickly tap into energy, memory, immunity, equilibrium and lower your sensitivity to pain.

When you're under chronic stress, however, increased levels of cortisol can wreak havoc by adversely affecting your brain, thyroid, blood sugar, bones, muscles, blood pressure, immunity and inflammation levels. Too much cortisol in the body, for instance, can result in foggy thinking, feeling run down, altered blood sugar levels and muscle discomfort. Cortisol can also affect your appetite.

Do personal trainers normally work with clients who are only free on weekends or during off-hours? What's typical in terms of when personal trainers are available?

Not at all. Unfortunately, many people have 9-5 jobs so the only time they can work out is early in the morning or in the evening. So it may be harder to schedule because those times are more in demand. Personally, as a full-time trainer, I would love more normal work hour appointments.

If someone has back problems, or other physical limitations, how can they lift weights safely, without getting hurt?

There are many other ways of working out without using weights. You need to heal and strengthen the injury or problem area before moving on to more challenging activities. This is where a trainer comes in handy, because they will know many ways to strengthen a muscle and they should also know your limits almost better than the client.

How should someone determine how many grams of protein and carbs they should be eating each day?

Well, textbook answer is 1.2-1.8 grams of protein per kilogram of body weight. 1 kg= 2.2lbs. Which turns out to not be as much as you think, a 6 oz. steak usually satisfies those numbers. It's not so important to worry about the specific amount as the kind of protein you are getting. Overdoing it can stress the adrenal glands, which can produce the stress hormone cortisol and actually sabotage your success.

You don't need a low-quality soy protein shake after your workout. Dark leafy greens have protein, certain grains like quinoa have protein as well. Then, of course, there are your meat, eggs, dairy, and nuts that are high in protein as well. Most people get enough from their diet. You want to get most of your carbs from vegetables and fruits.

You should avoid refined and processed grains and sugar like the plague. Think about what you're eating. Ask yourself, "how is this food going to help my body?" if you don't know, or know it won't help, walk away.

The new fad seems to be "buying organic". Is there any validity to eating organic food over non-organic food? What are the benefits and/or things to be aware of?

Conventional farming uses pesticides and genetically modified organisms. So buying organic you can at least avoid them. However like anything, there are pitfalls. We encourage you to know your local farmer and know how he produces your food. Then you have fresh, local, and likely organic foods.

The USDA must inspect a farm and the farmer must pay them, so many use organic methods, but don't get the USDA seal because of the cost. And then there are some certified organic farmers that probably cut corners. Know your farmer and eat time tested foods!

If someone reaches their fitness goals, should they still continue to work with a personal trainer?

That will depend on the person. Once you reach your goals, you will still need to do something to maintain your fitness level and expend some energy. If you can do that on your own, then maybe it's not necessary to keep a trainer. If, however, you need someone to tell you what to do and push you and keep you accountable, maybe keep meeting with your trainer once a week or so.

Hopefully your trainer has given you an education to take with you so you won't be dependent on them for the rest of your life. Find a trainer/teacher and learn.

Most experts seem to all agree that nuts are very healthy, but they seem to have a lot of fat in them. Won't eating high fat foods like nuts make it more difficult to lose weight?

Absolutely not. Its SUGAR & things that your body processes as sugar that make you gain weight, not fat. Fat is the body's preferred method of energy. You need to replace bad, stored fat with good fats like nuts and avocados. In addition, vitamins A,D,E and K (found in a lot of green veggies) are fat soluble which means they NEED fats to be transported throughout your body. Often times when you see foods that are low fat, they have removed some fat and replaced it with sugar, or worse, artificial sweeteners.

How important is nutrition if someone works out consistently?

Nutrition is extremely important. When you eat better, you will feel better in your workout. So in order to keep your workouts at their peak, you should eat the best you can. Once you've reached your goals, it is much easier to maintain without working out as much when you eat the way you should. We often say nutrition is 80% of the problem.

Why do people have such a hard time losing belly fat?

Belly fat is totally related to nutrition. Too much sugar, refined carbs, sodas and alcohol are usually the culprits of belly fat. You must cut out white flour and sugar to get rid of belly fat.

HOW TO CONTACT US

Terry Barga

Owner/Operator of Life Fitness Academy

Phone: 615-562-2633

Email: lifefitnessacademy@gmail.com

INTERVIEW WITH DERRICK SOBOTKA

6 GETTING A HELPING HAND

Since 1998, Barry's Bootcamp has been delivering "The Best Workout in the World" to a legendary following, including many celebrities. Our no-nonsense, results driven reputation may intimidate some newcomers, but they quickly discover that Barry's Bootcamp delivers an affordable, efficient and fun workout in a night club party environment that is nothing like the cliche boot camps found in every town.

What are some of the most common myths about nutrition?

I think the most common myth about nutrition is that it doesn't matter. In actuality your results are 60% in the kitchen. Without a positive relationship with food the workout is always going to suffer.

I like to describe the difference between a "diet" and "your diet" as two very different things. A "diet" is never going to work...it is a temporary fix for a long term issue. "Your diet" is your relationship with food. How often do you eat? What do you eat?

How does your relationship with food effect the results that you see from your workout. How do you need to change your relationship with food? Once you answer those questions and change the puzzle pieces that don't fit then you are on the road to a successful body.

What is a "drop set"?

A drop set is a commonly used term in exercise when you are attempting to reach total and complete failure in a specific muscle group. Let's take for example a bicep curl. You performing a bicep curl with a twenty pound set of weights to failure. When you reach that point of failure where you cannot perform another repetition you immediately drop down to a lower weight and continue that bicep curl. The philosophy is to take the specific muscle group to a point at which you might never have before.

If someone has a friend who is in good shape, who is willing to give them exercise advice, why is it still a good idea to hire a personal trainer?

There is no denying that a friend who is in good shape might know some great tips about exercising. A personal trainer, however, is educated and specialized in the finer things regarding exercise. Safety, perfect form, physical limitations and responsible exercise program design are all areas where a personal trainer is a master of. A personal trainer has the materials and know-how to track your progress. Education is power.

What are some tips to help people stick with an exercise program and not quit?

I have my clients do something a bit unorthodox to stay on track with their exercise program. I have my clients find a bathing suit, pair of skinny jeans, a dress, anything that they aspire to be able to fit in to. I have them purchase this article of clothing and hang it in their home where they will see it every single day. I also have them try it on or attempt to try it on once a month. Their goal is to fit into this article of clothing.

Almost every single time the client finally gets to the point to where they fit into this article of clothing. They met their goal!!! Sometimes that article of clothing ends up being too small!!! We have to celebrate our wins in life and seeing physical progress is always the most motivational.

How can people overcome junk food cravings?

I think that everyone struggles with cravings. We all have our little favorite snacks that we know we shouldn't have. It feels bad and sometimes feeling bad feels so good! I tend to have a fairly controversial way of doing things so what do I suggest? HAVE IT! Have a bite.

If you are craving cookies...have a bite. But just one bite. You would be shocked that just with one bite your craving will completely go away and then finish that hunger off with a positive food choice. Have a bite of that cookie and then move on to having a piece of fruit.

You are craving that cookie because your body is wanting something sweet. Give it what it wants...have the bite of the cookie and finish off that sweet tooth with the natural sugars from the fruit. Your body really doesn't know the difference. We have to trick it.

How does someone know if they're "over-training"?

There is a fine line between soreness due to training and soreness due to over training. Feeling a little bit sore from training is a perfectly normal feeling to have. Especially if you haven't exercised in a long time. Now if that soreness does not go away in a day or two you are over training. You shouldn't "hurt" from training you should feel the muscle responding to the stress you just put it under.

How does someone tone up and lose fat under their arms and around their triceps?

Interval cardiovascular work is always an important element of any workout program. It is very difficult, almost impossible, to just "spot treat" a specific problem area. The fat burning element of interval cardio is essential to reducing the fat from the problem areas. From that point you want to dive into resistance training.

If you want to tone up your arms you would transition into resistance training. Building lean muscle in any area is going to burn fat more efficiently when coupling it with your interval cardiovascular work. In the case of the arms. Always integrate the interval cardiovascular work to reduce the fat stores and then work with some isolated tricep work with movements like a tricep kickback, tricep pull-down, or an overhead tricep press.

What's the difference between "good carbs" and "bad carbs"?

There are carbs in almost anything you eat to a certain degree. The question is "what are they and what are they doing for you?" A bad carb is a carbohydrate that is or is made up of highly processed foods. These carbs will drastically spike your blood sugar.

You will also never really feel satisfied. You need some carbs for energy though. So how do we get them? Unrefined food. Take whole grains, vegetables, fruits or beans. All of these foods have carbohydrates in them and yet they are unrefined foods. Our body can identify them and use them to their fullest potential. We can use them completely.

What should people look out for when hiring a personal trainer?

Don't be afraid to do your homework. A good personal trainer should have their credentials in order to present to you. Are they certified, and not only that, are they certified through a reputable certification program. Ask them! Ask to see their certification or credentials. Also...what do their current or former clients have to say?

Don't be afraid to ask for references. A good trainer should be able to provide you with personal testimonies from clients who have used their professional services. Ask them about their experiences. Do your homework when you are putting your health in another person's hands.

What are some of the most common misconceptions that people have about hiring a personal trainer?

I think the most common misconception that I hear about hiring a personal trainer is that it is way too expensive. I generally like to put it into perspective for them. A personal trainer can run you anywhere from $75 per hour session all the way up to sometimes $200 per session. Even on the highest end of that pay scale a heart attack will cost you on average, including medication and doctor visits, roughly $50,000.00 per year for the rest of your life. I personally would much rather prevent that expense all together and pay the $75.00 to $200.00 as an investment toward my health.

HOW TO CONTACT US
Derrick Sobotka
Manager / Trainer Barry's Bootcamp
Website: www.barrysbootcamp.com
Phone: (619) 906-4455
Email: derrick@barrysbootcamp.com

INTERVIEW WITH IRV RUBENSTEIN

7 GETTING THE JOB DONE

Steps was founded in 1986 by myself and a fellow grad student in exercise science at Peabody College of Vanderbilt University, Nashville, TN. Our Intent was to introduce Nashville to a personal training facility where fitness professionals could rent time and space to provide their services to their own clients. In 1989 we opened our first facility and moved into our current location in 2000. Today about 20 trainers ply their trade as either independent operators (their own clientele) or independent contractors (training steps-derived clients).

What are the best foods that people should eat to gain energy and why are these foods so important?

Carbohydrates are the body's preferred source of energy with simpler versions most accessible shortly before and immediately after an exercise event/session and complex carbs for longer term energy storage and replenishment. For longer term exercise, fats are necessary; healthier fats are preferred, such as nuts and vegetable oils.

Is it better to lift weights with free weights or with weight machines? Why is one better than the other?

There are two ways to approach this question: For whom, and why? Without going into a dissertation on it, suffice it to say that there are times, clients, and exercises where machines are better or more apropos than free weights. While the latter are 'better' in that they more closely approximate the way our bodies have to actually stabilize a joint or joints in order to move another or others, and they do allow more 'functional' movement patterns overall, machines do serve a purpose.

For one, of all the major exercises – the pull from a high position – few people can do a pull up or chin up, so a lat pull will strengthen these most integral muscles for many sports and life activities – the forearm, biceps and lats. The other value to machines is for people who may require total stabilization and isolation at some phase of their training in order to strengthen muscles that will contribute to more functional movements.

Thus, for generally older clients with osteoarthritis of the knees or hips, machines allow one to condition muscles of the lower extremities without contributing to the already-worn out joints that would otherwise need to be done in closed-chain moves such as squats and lunges. For these and several other reasons I refuse to elevate one modality over another.

If someone needs to quickly lose a few pounds for a special occasion, what's the best way they can do this?

Cut calories. For the most part, Americans overeat as much as 25-50% of their caloric needs. I recommend cutting one-third of their total caloric intake from all their preferred food choices, even desserts. Doing so allows them to eat as they wish but cut calories in the process. If one has to cut more calories to lose weight prior to a special occasion, they could shift their macronutrient composition toward more proteins – but they need to drink more water to prevent the metabolic downsides from diminishing their energy and the effects of Ketosis that accompanies high protein diets.

What types of shoes should people wear when working out?

It depends on what kind of workout. If relatively static but needing support/cushioning, a cross trainer or even a low cost pair of K-Mart shoes will suffice. If you will be doing movements such as agility or plyometrics, you may need a different shoe to accommodate the surface, type of moves, and speeds at which you're doing them.

Can someone use a personal trainer to help them rehabilitate from a sports injury? How would this be handled?

Yes. But I would suggest one seeks a trainer with a more advanced education or more years of experience. Getting a referral from a doctor or therapist will provide some assurance of qualifications and understanding of the nature of the problem and a hint of experience with other clients who'd seen him/her.

Is it possible to lose fat and gain muscle at the same time? If so, how can this be done effectively?

Clearly this is more possible for males, and for younger people than older people. Studies do not show that middle age women can readily build muscle – 1-2# is what many short-term studies show. (Few studies of this nature have gone beyond 6 months so it's hard to say what those numbers look like.) Losing fat is best accomplished by cutting calories, plus cardio exercise at moderate or high intensities.

Adding large body movement exercises such as squats, lunges, chest presses, overhead presses, pull downs and rows, plus many of the 'fuctional' and Olympic exercises, ensures greater caloric burn plus greater muscle accretion if, and I do mean if, the resistances are high enough to generate protein accretion. Many older folks are not willing to work that hard but if they do, they can build some muscle. It helps to be male, however.

How soon, after someone starts a diet and exercise program, should they start to see results, to know if their diet and exercise program is working?

It's a matter of what results one is trying to achieve. If we're talking weight loss or size loss, it could be 4-8 weeks before those results show up. If it's strength or function, it could be within 2-4 weeks. If it's definition or hypertrophy, it could be 8-16 weeks. But if it's to feel and move better, it could be almost immediately. Some people simply need to start moving more to feel better.

If someone is a heavy smoker, should their workout routine be adjusted at all? If so, how?

It depends on age and other health factors. Young heavy smokers, while at greater risk than non-smokers of similar activity status – presumably sedentary – can be pushed pretty hard, almost as hard as a previously sedentary person. Older heavy smokers are likely to have co-morbidities such as hypertension, heart disease, etc. and should be regarded from that perspective rather than just their smoking habit.

Is there any truth to the claim that exercise can help improve brain function and/or mental focus? If yes, how?

Yes, definitely. Several studies published in 2012 have demonstrated improved cognitive function and memory in those who do regular cardio exercise; some second-half of 2012 have shown similar though lesser benefits from resistance training programs. Those few that have combined the two modalities have shown benefits closer to those of cardio-only programs.

As to how these occur, the first thoughts have to do with blood flow overall but obviously to the brain. Secondary mechanisms are hypothesized to come through neurological relationships with the musculoskeletal movements that all forms of exercise demand. In fact, these may be more a factor for benefits from a resistance training program as the moves are more diverse, multi-directional, multi-factorial – Think balance and stability both of specific joints as well as the body itself – and usually more demanding – think intensity at the end of a set of series of sets, which requires mental input. There are probably some hormonal and metabolic inputs to the benefits of exercise, from insulin levels to blood sugar control, too.

Can couples or groups of people workout with a personal trainer at the same time?

Of course. Is it possible to be as observant of new clients especially while teaching or performing more complex moves? If treated properly, and taught progressively, yes, although many instructors fail to take into consideration the variety of limitations and needs of all the participants in a class format. Thus, If one's needs are greater, the smaller the group, the better for the client.

HOW TO CONTACT US
Irv Rubenstein
President/CEO of STEPS, Inc.
Phone: 615- 269-8855
Email: irvrube@gmail.com

INTERVIEW WITH DANNY KACZMAREK

8 EATING YOUR WAY TO A HEALTHIER BODY

What can thin people do to build muscle?

Our genetic structure (phenotype) and dimensions are determined by the genetics that have been handed down to us. In terms of muscle or amount of muscle present without any training stimulation, this is called (myostatin gene loci). So the genetics you have are the genetics you have.

We typically call these people "hard gainers". But over time as you reach muscle maturity and your metabolic rate slows a little bit you will be surprised at how much muscle you can put on if you really work hard at it and stay consistent. Remember that this is a lifestyle, nothing happens too quickly.

Maximizing your genetic output requires the correct training protocols and what I call a genetically balanced diet that causes your body to maximize it's potential within. It has to do with certain nutrients influencing your genetics to make more muscle and burn more fat. This is the study of Epi-Genetics and or Nutrigenomics, the influence that nutrients have on genetic expression.

This can take years of trial and error. But now there are genetic test kits available that can reveal to you how much aerobic training you need compared to the anaerobic training you need. They can also tell you what the percentages of your carbohydrate, protein, and fat intake should be. These tests take out all the guesswork saving you time and money. You literally get a road map that tells you exactly what you need in these ratios to maximize your genetic potential!

What are some factors that impact people's metabolism?

This is a loaded question. Many books could be written on this because our overall metabolism is affected by so many factors. Metabolism is the sum total of our organ systems' function, both internal (physiological) and external (phenotypic) behaviors, predicated on our genetics and the relationship of Epigenetic stimulation or inhibition on our genetic "footprint." Therefore, our Metabolism is determined by many internal and external environmental variables.

Here are a few points

1- Stress! That's number one! Excessive stress can wreak havoc on ones metabolic rate. Like heart rate, glucose levels, sleep disorders, and excessive pain and inflammation in body tissues. People can tend to react differently to various stressors as well. Some gain weight by eating too much (i.e. comfort food) and some lose weight as they tend to eat less during times of stress.

2- Exercise (positive or good stress) can have a positive impact on our metabolism as it has the ability to increase our metabolic rate so we are able to burn more calories, even at rest, while recovering from workout to workout. This especially has to do with the muscle resistance types of exercises by using your own body weight, free weights or machines.

3- Excessive toxicities or too much exposure to various pollutants can cause the body to be extra stressed and over loads and stagnates the various detoxification systems and pathways, especially in the liver. This can slow you down!

What can people do to stay motivated, after they've started a workout program?

Constantly change up your workout routine or it can get stale pretty quick. Try various types of training classes like boot camps, martial arts, kick boxing, zumba, weight training, etc... Also try looking at exercise videos for new ideas and insights on how to train certain ways and certain body parts. This will keep things from getting monotonous and can be highly motivational as well.

Can sit-ups help people lose belly fat? Why do some people do thousands of sit-ups and they still don't lose any belly fat?

Losing body fat comes from a complete body loss of adipose tissue. THERE IS NO SUCH THING AS SPOT REDUCING! Your body needs to create heat. This is called thermogenesis or becoming thermogenic. Your body runs faster and hotter creating heat because you have done things to speed up your metabolic rate like exercising and eating sensibly according to your genetic design. This in turn will help you burn more calories at rest which then allows the body to free up it's fat storage to be burned off for energy purposes.

If someone has a personal trainer, do they also need a nutritionist? What are the differences between a personal trainer and a nutritionist?

They don't necessarily need a nutritionist but it couldn't hurt that's for sure. In my experience I knew from day one that nutrition had everything to do with health and fitness and wellness. You cannot maximize your genetic potential without the correct nutritional intake. This is why I decided to become an N.D. (Naturopathic Doctor). This is a doctor of natural medicine using various types of nutritional elements to feed the body in such a way so as to heal faster from training, sickness and disease. Again, tapping into your genetic potential.

Trainer- One who teaches you how to train your body to become more fit and strong using all kinds of exercise principles.

Nutritionist- One who teaches you how to feed and hydrate your body in order to maximize results.

What is "core strength"?

"The strength and the power of your body from the belly button out". It is the foundation of true strength and fitness. Moving our limbs comes from the trunk of your body. (Rectus abdominus, obliques, transverse abdominus, spinal erectors, serratus, and every muscle/tendon attachment that connects to your spine and upper pelvis are your core muscles that need to be trained.

This could also include some other pelvic attachments as well. Just about every human kinetic movement requires the core (trunk) to be engaged. A strong core leads to stronger limbs and a stronger you in every facet of exercise. Your core is the key!

Why is it better to eat more frequent, smaller meals throughout the day than less frequent larger meals?

Smaller more frequent meals are easier for your digestive system to break down and assimilate into our bloodstream. When this can be done efficiently your G.E.T or gastric emptying time (when food leaves the stomach into the small intestine) speeds up slightly and elevates our metabolic rate. Hence, creating that thermogenic (heat) effect we spoke of earlier.

Larger meals do the opposite by placing too much burden on the digestive system which in turn, will slow you down and your metabolic rate. A fast metabolism burns fat and builds muscle. A slow metabolic rate burns muscle and builds fat.

How often should someone workout with a personal trainer?

As much as they can as long as they are recovering from their training sessions in a timely manner. That's the most important thing. Finances always play a major role as well. But typically it's anywhere from 2 to 4 times a week training.

Every day, there seems to be a new "health food" product on the grocery store shelves. How can people tell if a food item is really healthy or not?

Read, read, read and study, study, study. There is SO MUCH out there it can be really confusing. You have to educate yourself to a certain degree. The one thing about this industry is that it can unfortunately deceive a lot of people just to make a buck. Sad, but true. So here is a list of some nutrients that absolutely work because they are cell receptor compatible. That means they are friendly to your cells and relatively easy to digest and absorb.

1-Probiotics. Healthy gut bacteria (flora) that play a huge role in our immune function, controlling body inflammation, and breaking down nutrients to their smallest sub-units so they can be utilized by the cells of the body. Books can be written on what gut flora can do!

What is a healthy amount of weight to lose each week? Why is it a bad idea to lose more weight than this each week?

Depending on an individual's metabolic balance (homeostatic platform) and physical and physiological health, weight loss should probably not be more than the 1-2% of an individual's "ideal," genetically predetermined body weight. 2 to 6 lbs. per week should be ideal. Anymore then that can lead to an increased stress response in the body that can affect glucose levels which in turn stresses the body even more on multiple levels.

Our metabolic rate can only go so fast in terms of dropping body fat weight. There's a metabolic timer on each cell of our body that cannot be pushed too hard before it becomes dysfunctional. People tend to drop their calories too low for too long of a time. There has to be that balance of calories up and calories down. Too much emphasis is placed on the amount of calories instead of the QUALITY of the calories you take in.

What happens at the initial appointment with a personal trainer?

It tends to be a meet and greet and sometimes a workout assessment to look for strengths and weaknesses in the individual. Compatibility is a major issue when it comes to personal training. Because it's personal, a client should feel comfortable with the trainer they choose. This leads to far better results because psychological factors and expectations are being met.

There seems to be a lot of talk about these "cleansing diets", where people just drink lemon juice with cayenne pepper and some sort of syrup for 30 or more days. Is this safe and/or healthy? Why or why not?

Cleanses can be safe for some, and not safe for others. This is an actual fasting type of cleanse. Fasting can actually be incredibly beneficial for a person because it increases the speed of all the detox pathways in the body. When you drop calories like this program does, the body can concentrate on cleaning house because you are taking the digestive process out of the way so the body can now spend it's dominant energy on the elimination processes instead. All of this depends on the state of health an individual is in when they start this program.

I would start by decreasing caloric intake over a 5-day period before starting this type of cleanse. This will help your body adjust to the sudden change in caloric intake once the cleanse has started. I would only do this for 7 to 10 days to start to see how your body reacts.

After this initial personal assessment, about a month or so you can experiment by going longer than the 7 to 10 day time frame. Again, if you detox too rapidly it can place too much stress on the body which can lead to unwanted problems like excessive headaches, rashes, low energy, and brain fog to name a few. I personally like vegetable juice fasting. If you own a juicer I recommend this recipe although there are hundreds of recipes out there:

1 Apple

4 Celery stalks

1 Cucumber

1 inch slice of fresh Ginger

1 Red or yellow bell pepper

2 to 3 leaflets of Red chard (if available)

This is a low sugar but sweet tasting drink that is anti-oxidant loaded that satisfies, detoxifies, and increases blood flow for you at the same time. I cannot over emphasize enough that eating and drinking the "colors of the rainbow" is probably the healthiest thing you can do for your body!

HOW TO CONTACT US

Danny Kaczmarek

Website: www.innovativefitness.info

Website: www.biocencestore.com

Phone: 214-449-6863

Email: dtex777@me.com

9 TIPS TO PICK THE BEST WORKOUT PROGRAM

Poise Health & Fitness offers personal fitness training to help you live a life of balance, strength, and stability. Our goal is to give you the tools, education, confidence and motivation you need to make health and fitness part of your lifestyle rather than a passing phase. We combine functional strength, flexibility, cardiovascular fitness, stability training, and nutrition coaching to help you achieve your goals and realize your potential.

Is it a good idea to walk or run with weights? Will this produce results more quickly?

It's never a good idea to hold weights while running or walking because it compromises your posture and form. Holding weights while running, for example, causes the shoulders and upper back to slump forward, which puts greater strain on your spine and neck. You'll likely decrease performance as a result. For faster results mixing cardio and weights, opt for circuit training instead.

If someone has been a "yo-yo dieter" their entire lives, how can a personal trainer help people like this?

A personal trainer can help identify the key issues at play with a yo-yo dieter. Perhaps it's psychological, or perhaps it's purely that the client always resorts to a strict diet as a last resort, which never works in the long-term. It's a personal trainer's job to identify, educate, and find the means for making good health a lifestyle for each client.

What is "body fat percentage"? How does this differ from "body mass index"?

Body fat percentage is a measurement of total adipose (fatty) tissue in the body. Body mass index, on the other hand, is an estimate of body fat based on height and weight. The methods used for measuring body fat percentage are ultimately more reliable than those used for body mass index. BMI does not take into account, for example, someone who is a body builder and has a significant amount of lean muscle weight. On a BMI chart, it would categorize this person as obese.

What exactly does a personal trainer do?

A personal trainer acts as a coach, partner, educator and motivator to those looking to make a difference in their lives through fitness and health. Trainers design a program customized to each client's goals and abilities in order to help them succeed in reaching their potential. A trainer also acts as someone the client has to be accountable to.

What is a medical release and when is it necessary?

A medical release form is usually filled out by either the client or client's physician, and signed by their physician, to give consent to the trainer to move ahead with designing a workout program. This usually comes into play with clients who have a history of medical issues, or in the elderly population.

Why is it so important to drink water and how much water should people drink each day?

Water aids in the process of every bodily function and is vital for producing energy in the body, so if you want a good workout you should make sure you're properly hydrated both before, during and after.

The requirement is different for everyone based on daily activity, weight and environment, but as a general rule I tell my male clients to drink around 128 ounces a day, and females to drink 88 ounces.

Is it unhealthy to eat a vegetarian or vegan diet that has no meat or dairy?

As long as you are getting enough lean protein, iron, and calcium, it's perfectly healthy to live a vegetarian or vegan diet. If I see a client who has obvious iron deficiencies, however, I encourage them to consider the flexitarian diet, which simply means eating less meat than typical diets (perhaps meat only once a week).

How do people measure their heart rate?

They can measure it manually, by placing their fingers over a pulse point (usually neck or wrist) and counting each beat for 10 seconds, then multiply that number by 6 to get their heart rate beat per minute. Or they can measure using a heart rate monitor, which are most accurate when a chest strap is worn.

How should the diet of someone who's looking to build muscle differ from the diet of someone who's looking to lose weight?

Someone who's wanting to shed pounds needs to consume fewer calories than they take in. A pound of fat is 3500 calories, so to lose a pound a week they need to have a calorie deficit of 3500 over the course of the week. Someone looking to build muscle, on the other hand, will need a surplus of calories, made up mostly of lean quality proteins and healthy carbohydrates.

Is it better for someone to workout at home or at a gym with their personal trainer? What are the pros and cons to each?

Whichever means a person will be able to commit to is the best. For many of my clients they train with me and have for years because they just won't do it on their own and they know it, so they dedicate time in their schedule for meeting with me. For others who are diligent and self-disciplined, working out at home can be just as effective. The pros to working with a trainer are extra accountability and motivation, a customized workout routine, and someone to keep your form in check for optimal results. The cons are it's expensive. The pros to working out at home are convenience, privacy, and affordability. The cons are there is room for error in form if the person is new to working out, and motivation may wane if no one else is there to make you accountable.

If someone has a favorite food that they could never give up forever, what do you suggest?

So don't! My clients and I live by the 80/20 rule. 80% of the time eat well, meaning healthy, clean and as fresh as possible. 20% of the time you can indulge in your favorite food. This may come down to 80% of the week you eat healthy and 20% you splurge, or 80% of each day you eat healthy and you have one treat (usually a snack) that makes you feel you're not giving up what you love.

What should people look out for when joining a gym?

Make sure it's in a convenient location for you, so many people join up thinking they'll make the trek each day, but convenience is so important for long-term success. Also interview the trainers to find the right fit for you. Someone who primarily trains body builders is not the best choice for a client looking to shed pounds and tone up.

Their personality must also mesh with yours. Check for cleanliness of the equipment, how the staff treats customers and each other, and what the renewal terms are. Many of my clients have been burned by big-box gyms who renew memberships and alter contracts without notifying the customer. Also, if you're interested in group classes make sure they offer them at times that work with your schedule, and if day care is needed make sure you get a good vibe from the people who will be watching your children.

HOW TO CONTACT US
Crystal Potter
Owner of Poise Health & Fitness
Website: www.poisefitness.net
Email: crystalthomas@poisefitness.net

INTERVIEW WITH STEVE & TORI BRADFORD

10 A CERTAIN WAY DOES HELP

Center-Fit was founded by two personal trainers, a husband and wife team, Steve & Tori Bradford. We now have turned our goal focused personal training into small group exercise classes including kettlebells, boxing, yoga, zumba, and bootcamps.

Is it true that it's bad to eat too much fruit because of all of the sugar it contains?

While fruit does contain a lot of sugar grams technically, the sugar comes from a natural and unprocessed source (fructose). We believe that the healthiest foods you can eat come from the ground and were made by God and not man. So no, fruit is not "bad" because of the sugar, however the quantity is important. For example, I wouldn't sit down to eat 4 bananas at once, but 1 banana while high in sugar is perfectly suitable and even nourishing to the body.

Is it true that exercise and a healthy diet can help reduce the chance of developing diabetes? If this is true, how can exercise and/or a good nutrition plan help prevent diabetes?

Yes it is true that nourishing nutrition and purposeful movement can help prevent the risk of developing Type 2 Diabetes. Diabetes is a disease based on the body's inability to efficiently utilize blood sugar and recognize insulin. It has been proven that the types of foods we eat affect our blood sugars because of the speed at which the food is broken down. Foods are considered to be "high-glycemic" when the blood sugar spikes after the food has been ingested. These foods are normally carbohydrates that have been highly processed and refined so the body breaks them down quickly. The more often these foods are eaten, the body becomes bogged down with these high levels of blood sugars and it can cause problems for the pancreas creating an insensitivity to the body's insulin thus creating the onset of diabetes. Exercise also plays a role in managing blood sugar because muscles use blood sugar as energy, so if a person does not purposefully move like in exercise the body does not use energy a.k.a. blood sugar. Purposeful movement creates an environment for the muscles to call on blood sugar to be used as energy, thus using any extra blood sugar that the body may have in the blood stream.

What's the difference between "aerobic" and "anaerobic" exercises?

It's the difference between a marathon runner and a sprinter. A marathon runner, similar to aerobic exercise, uses long steady oxygen, where as anaerobic exercise like the sprinter uses quick bursts of energy/oxygen and would be unable to sustain that level of intensity for a long period of time.

Are certain types of cardio workouts better than others?

Yes absolutely! A lot of research points to interval trainings being a much more efficient form of cardio workouts that maximizes total caloric burn, as well as burns a higher percentage of those calories coming from fat.

Who should the average person talk to about which exercise program would be best for them?

We recommend speaking with someone that has certifications in the area they are training in from a reputable organization. The fitness industry is full of trainers that only took a test online and may or may not have any real experience with movement patterns or health. Anyone can give you a good workout that burns calories, but a true trainer will have knowledge on how the body SHOULD move and why.

Does a person have to check with their doctor before beginning a workout program with a personal trainer?

It is always recommended that a person check with their regular physician before beginning any new exercise program. While exercise and purposeful movement is great for the body, many people need to take it slow at the beginning.

Is it a good idea to workout when feeling mentally stressed? Why or why not?

Purposeful movement in the form of a workout routine can be extremely beneficial for reducing mental and emotional stress. There are many reasons for this including the increase in endorphins that are released, the feeling of accomplishment, and of course achieving goals. I believe the main reason for this is called meditation in movement which is the concept that while you are focusing on the movement or exercise at hand, you are no longer focusing on the stresses of your day or life, therefore reducing any stress that you may have been dealing with before you started your workout.

In addition to working out, what are some of the most beneficial activities to participate in and why are these activities so beneficial/healthy?

We recommend that everyone live an active lifestyle. It's great to have a regular workout routine, but the most important aspect of a healthy life is consistency in movement. These activities can include the whole family and should be fun like playing sports, hiking, biking, etc. Including these activities in your daily life will be beneficial for your family and their health.

How long should a personal training session last?

Most personal training sessions last either 30 minutes or 60 minutes. We utilize hard style kettle bells in most of our training sessions which are very efficient tools and workouts can be completed in less time with the same caloric and fat burn as in traditional workouts.

How do people get rid of loose skin after weight loss?

Well the only natural way to get rid of loose skin is to lose the weight slow and steady so that the body has time to adapt to this loss in fat. The younger a person is the easier this process is because the elasticity of the skin is still very strong, as a person ages they begin to lose this elasticity.

What are some tips that people should keep in mind, for practicing good form during their workouts?

We are big advocates of maintaining good form in their workouts, not just because their workout will be more efficient, but because they will reduce the risk of overuse injuries to their joints and tendons. Some good tips would include not doing something if it hurts, workout barefoot so you can feel the ground on all four corners of your feet, keep the knees over the ankles, hips over knees, shoulders over hips, and chin up.

Do people have to join the gym that their personal trainer belongs to, in order to hire them?

This policy changes with each gym, so you should check with your trainer. Many trainers are available to train in your home, or even in a small studio. In my experience, the best trainers have their own studios or work for themselves, so you should seek them out in your area.

HOW TO CONTACT US

Steve & Tori Bradford
Owners, Personal and Group Trainers of Center-Fit
Website: center-fit.com
Phone: 630-449-7331
Email: info@center-fit.com

CONCLUSION

Congratulations on making it to the end of this book! We hope that you realize and appreciate the immense level of real world knowledge that you've just acquired. The one thing you may be feeling, at this point, is a bit of "information overload", due to the many tips, pieces of advice, and strategies that are jammed into this book. If you are feeling a bit overwhelmed from everything you've just learned, allow us to offer you one final piece of advice: Take a day to let your brain absorb all of the information you just learned. As they say: "Sleep on it". If you attempt to try and remember and implement everything you just learned, your efforts may tend to be scattered and a bit unorganized. Instead, take a day off from the information. If you do this, you're likely to find that you develop a sense of clarity and a better perspective on the information.

Once you've taken a day to allow yourself to re-focus in this way, we encourage you to slowly go back through the book, writing down the actionable information that you intend to implement. Simply reading and understanding the information is not enough. By writing down the information that you plan on implementing, it will allow you to put a clear plan of action into place for yourself.

As you go through the information, don't worry about the order in which you write things down. The first thing to do is to just get the information down on paper. There are many great strategies and tips within this book, but the goal here is for you to extract the exact advice that you will be taking action on. Don't worry if you are unsure about whether or not you will be taking immediate action on certain advice. Just write down everything that you may possibly take action on.

Once you've compiled this list of action steps and "maybe action steps", begin to prioritize this list. In other words, re-write the list with the actions that you know you're going to take at the top of the list and the action items that you may not take action on towards the bottom of the list. By organizing your list in this way, you will be able to build a practical, useable to-do list, from the information you learned in this book. Once you've done this, you will be in an excellent position to start taking focused steps, with clarity and purpose.

As we mentioned at the beginning of this book, most peddlers or fitness products and information hope that you keep buying their stuff. In keeping with the rebellious nature of this book, we encourage you to stop buying more fitness stuff and start implementing what you just learned in this book! Just as we have shared interviews with real world experts who actually do what they talk about in this book, it is our hope that you, as the reader, will take real world action on the information you've learned here.

Wishing you all the best in your action-taking, fitness and nutrition endeavors!

www.ingramcontent.com/pod-product-compliance
Lightning Source LLC
Chambersburg PA
CBHW070540290526
45790CB00002B/574